LOW GLYCEMIC INDEX DIABETIC RECIPES

RECIPES

Healthy, Delicious Meals for Managing Blood Sugar

Dr Lily Morgan

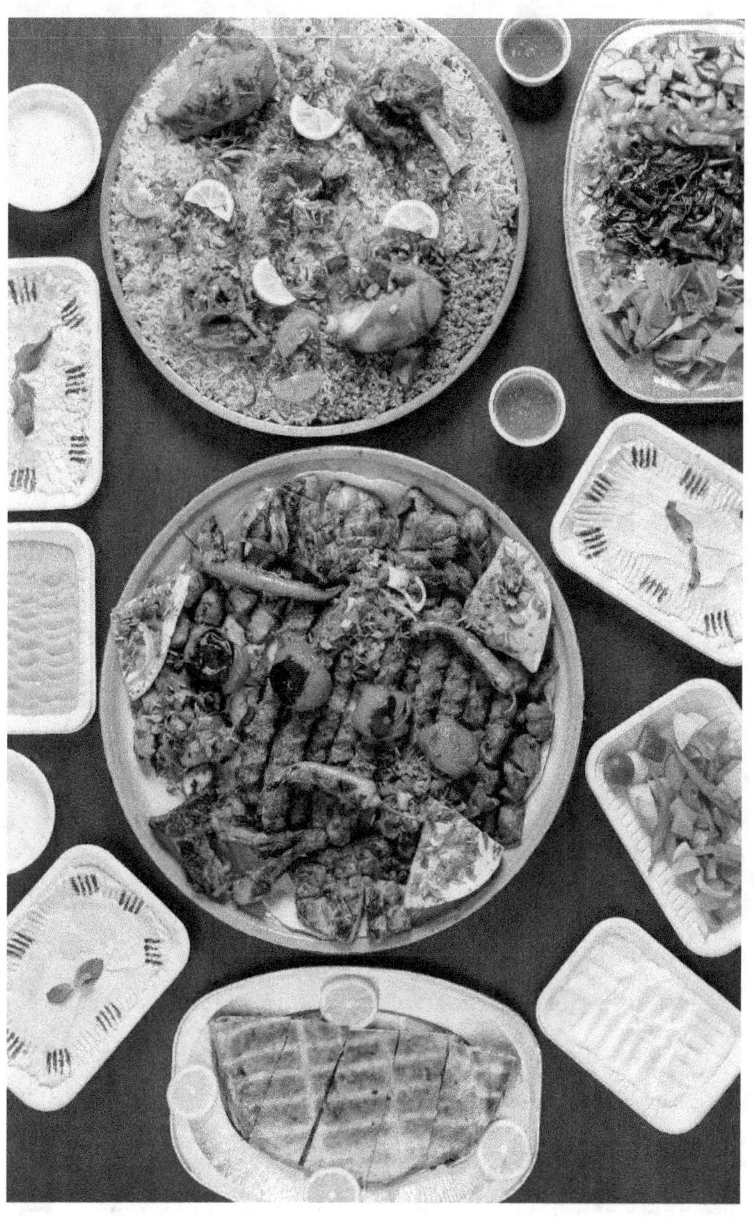

TABLE OF CONTENTS

Chapter 5: Snacks and Appetizers 57

INTRODUCTION

The Glycemic Index (GI) is a valuable tool for individuals with diabetes, offering insight into how different foods affect blood sugar levels. While the GI is a scientific concept, it's important to grasp its practical implications for managing diabetes through diet.

At its core, the Glycemic Index is a ranking system that assigns numerical values to carbohydrate-containing foods based on how quickly they raise blood sugar levels. Foods with a high GI are rapidly digested and absorbed, leading to quick spikes in blood sugar. Conversely, low-GI foods are digested more slowly, resulting in gradual, steady increases in blood sugar.

Understanding this concept is essential for diabetics because it enables them to make informed food choices. By opting for foods with a low GI, individuals can help stabilize their blood sugar levels, reducing the need for insulin or other medications.

However, it's important to note that the GI isn't the sole factor to consider when managing diabetes through diet. Portion control, overall carbohydrate intake, and the quality of carbohydrates matter as well. A balanced diet that combines low-GI foods with lean proteins, healthy fats, and plenty of fiber is the key to long-term blood sugar control.

Practical strategies for incorporating low-GI foods into your diet include choosing whole grains over refined grains, favoring non-starchy vegetables, and incorporating legumes and nuts. Additionally, it's beneficial to pair carbohydrates with protein and healthy fats to slow digestion further.

In summary, comprehending the Glycemic Index is a vital step in managing diabetes through diet. It empowers individuals to make healthier food choices, ultimately contributing to better blood sugar control. Yet, it should be seen as part of a broader dietary strategy that encompasses portion control and overall nutrient balance. By combining these principles, individuals with diabetes can enjoy a healthier, more stable lifestyle.

Chapter 1: 30-Day Meal Plan

Week 1

Day 1:

- Breakfast: Scrambled Egg Whites with Spinach and Tomatoes
- Lunch: Grilled Chicken Salad
- Dinner: Baked Salmon with Dill
- Snacks: Guacamole with Veggie Sticks
- Dessert: Berry and Yogurt Parfait

Day 2:

- Breakfast: Greek Yogurt Parfait with Berries
- Lunch: Lentil Soup
- Dinner: Chicken and Broccoli Stir-Fry
- Snacks: Roasted Chickpeas
- Dessert: Dark Chocolate-Covered Strawberries

Day 3:

- Breakfast: Oatmeal with Nuts and Berries
- Lunch: Quinoa Salad

- Dinner: Spinach and Mushroom Stuffed Pork Tenderloin
- Snacks: Cottage Cheese and Pineapple
- Dessert: Greek Yogurt with Honey and Walnuts

Day 4:

- Breakfast: Veggie Omelette
- Lunch: Tuna Lettuce Wraps
- Dinner: Grilled Vegetable Plate
- Snacks: Edamame
- Dessert: Sugar-Free Apple Crisp

Day 5:

- Breakfast: Whole Grain Pancakes
- Lunch: Turkey and Avocado Wrap
- Dinner: Beef and Snow Pea Stir-Fry
- Snacks: Hummus and Whole Grain Crackers
- Dessert: Baked Pears with Cinnamon

Day 6:

- Breakfast: Chia Seed Pudding
- Lunch: Spinach and Chickpea Salad

- Dinner: Lemon Herb Baked Tilapia

- Snacks: Greek Salad Skewers

- Dessert: Avocado Chocolate Mousse

Day 7:

- Breakfast: Breakfast Burrito

- Lunch: Cucumber and Hummus Sandwich

- Dinner: Turkey and Quinoa Stuffed Bell Peppers

- Snacks: Avocado Slices with Salsa

- Dessert: Chia Seed Chocolate Pudding

Week 2

Day 8:

- Breakfast: Almond Butter Toast

- Lunch: Salmon and Asparagus

- Dinner: Spaghetti Squash with Pesto

- Snacks: Deviled Eggs

- Dessert: Coconut Macaroons

Day 9:

- Breakfast: Smoothie Bowl

- Lunch: Spinach and Feta Stuffed Chicken Breast

- Dinner: Cabbage and Turkey Sauté

- Snacks: Zucchini Chips

- Dessert: Raspberry Sorbet

Day 10:

- Breakfast: Avocado Toast

- Lunch: Black Bean and Quinoa Bowl

- Dinner: Baked Cod with Asparagus

- Snacks: Cucumber Rolls with Cream Cheese

- Dessert: Almond and Blueberry Bites

Day 11:

- Breakfast: Cottage Cheese Pancakes

- Lunch: Shrimp and Vegetable Stir-Fry

- Dinner: Chicken and Zucchini Skewers

- Snacks: Caprese Skewers

- Dessert: Lemon Poppy Seed Cake

Day 12:

- Breakfast: Quinoa Porridge

- Lunch: Egg Salad Lettuce Wraps

- Dinner: Quinoa and Black Bean Stuffed Peppers

- Snacks: Mixed Nuts
- Dessert: Peanut Butter Protein Balls

Day 13:

- Breakfast: Veggie Frittata
- Lunch: Cauliflower Rice Bowl
- Dinner: Seared Tofu with Vegetables
- Snacks: Seaweed Snacks
- Dessert: Vanilla and Almond Milkshake

Day 14:

- Breakfast: Breakfast Quiche
- Lunch: Caprese Salad
- Dinner: Shrimp Scampi
- Snacks: Baked Sweet Potato Fries
- Dessert: Pumpkin Pie Smoothie

Week 3

Day 15:

- Breakfast: Berry Smoothie
- Lunch: Sweet Potato and Black Bean Quesadilla
- Dinner: Vegetable Curry

- Snacks: Mini Meatballs with Dipping Sauce
- Dessert: Banana Walnut Ice Cream

Day 16:

- Breakfast: Scrambled Egg Whites with Spinach and Tomatoes
- Lunch: Grilled Chicken Salad
- Dinner: Baked Salmon with Dill
- Snacks: Guacamole with Veggie Sticks
- Dessert: Berry and Yogurt Parfait

Day 17:

- Breakfast: Greek Yogurt Parfait with Berries
- Lunch: Lentil Soup
- Dinner: Chicken and Broccoli Stir-Fry
- Snacks: Roasted Chickpeas
- Dessert: Dark Chocolate-Covered Strawberries

Day 18:

- Breakfast: Oatmeal with Nuts and Berries
- Lunch: Quinoa Salad

- Dinner: Spinach and Mushroom Stuffed Pork Tenderloin
- Snacks: Cottage Cheese and Pineapple
- Dessert: Greek Yogurt with Honey and Walnuts

Day 19:

- Breakfast: Veggie Omelette
- Lunch: Tuna Lettuce Wraps
- Dinner: Grilled Vegetable Plate
- Snacks: Edamame
- Dessert: Sugar-Free Apple Crisp

Day 20:

- Breakfast: Whole Grain Pancakes
- Lunch: Turkey and Avocado Wrap
- Dinner: Beef and Snow Pea Stir-Fry
- Snacks: Hummus and Whole Grain Crackers
- Dessert: Baked Pears with Cinnamon

Day 21:

- Breakfast: Chia Seed Pudding
- Lunch: Spinach and Chickpea Salad

- Dinner: Lemon Herb Baked Tilapia

- Snacks: Greek Salad Skewers

- Dessert: Avocado Chocolate Mousse

Week 4

Day 22:

- Breakfast: Breakfast Burrito

- Lunch: Cucumber and Hummus Sandwich

- Dinner: Turkey and Quinoa Stuffed Bell Peppers

- Snacks: Avocado Slices with Salsa

- Dessert: Chia Seed Chocolate Pudding

Day 23:

- Breakfast: Almond Butter Toast

- Lunch: Salmon and Asparagus

- Dinner: Spaghetti Squash with Pesto

- Snacks: Deviled Eggs

- Dessert: Coconut Macaroons

Day 24:

- Breakfast: Smoothie Bowl

- Lunch: Spinach and Feta Stuffed Chicken Breast

- Dinner: Cabbage and Turkey Sauté
- Snacks: Zucchini Chips
- Dessert: Raspberry Sorbet

Day 25:

- Breakfast: Avocado Toast
- Lunch: Black Bean and Quinoa Bowl
- Dinner: Baked Cod with Asparagus
- Snacks: Cucumber Rolls with Cream Cheese
- Dessert: Almond and Blueberry Bites

Day 26:

- Breakfast: Cottage Cheese Pancakes
- Lunch: Shrimp and Vegetable Stir-Fry
- Dinner: Chicken and Zucchini Skewers
- Snacks: Caprese Skewers
- Dessert: Lemon Poppy Seed Cake

Day 27:

- Breakfast: Quinoa Porridge
- Lunch: Egg Salad Lettuce Wraps
- Dinner: Quinoa and Black Bean Stuffed Peppers

- Snacks: Mixed Nuts
- Dessert: Peanut Butter Protein Balls

Day 28:

- Breakfast: Veggie Frittata
- Lunch: Cauliflower Rice Bowl
- Dinner: Seared Tofu with Vegetables
- Snacks: Seaweed Snacks
- Dessert: Vanilla and Almond Milkshake

Day 29:

- Breakfast: Breakfast Quiche
- Lunch: Caprese Salad
- Dinner: Shrimp Scampi
- Snacks: Baked Sweet Potato Fries
- Dessert: Pumpkin Pie Smoothie

Day 30:

- Breakfast: Berry Smoothie
- Lunch: Sweet Potato and Black Bean Quesadilla
- Dinner: Vegetable Curry
- Snacks: Mini Meatballs with Dipping Sauce

- Dessert: Banana Walnut Ice Cream

You've now completed a comprehensive 30-day meal plan with a wide variety of low glycemic index diabetic-friendly recipes. This plan should help you manage your diabetes while enjoying delicious and nutritious meals.

Chapter 2: Breakfast Recipes

Welcome to the delightful world of healthy breakfasts! This chapter is dedicated to ensuring your mornings start with a burst of flavor and nutrition. From creamy parfaits to savory omelettes, you'll find a variety of options to satisfy your taste buds while keeping your blood sugar in check.

Scrambled Egg Whites with Spinach and Tomatoes

Ingredients:

- 4 egg whites
- 1 cup fresh spinach
- 1/2 cup cherry tomatoes, halved
- Salt and pepper to taste

Instructions:

1. Whisk the egg whites until frothy.
2. Heat a non-stick pan and add spinach and tomatoes.
3. Pour in the egg whites and scramble until cooked.
4. Season with salt and pepper. Serve hot.

Greek Yogurt Parfait with Berries

Ingredients:

- 1 cup Greek yogurt
- 1/2 cup mixed berries (strawberries, blueberries, raspberries)
- 2 tablespoons honey
- 1/4 cup granola (optional)

Instructions:

1. In a glass, layer Greek yogurt, berries, and honey.
2. Repeat the layers.
3. Top with granola for added crunch. Enjoy!

Oatmeal with Nuts and Berries

Ingredients:

- 1/2 cup rolled oats
- 1 cup almond milk
- 1/4 cup mixed nuts (almonds, walnuts)
- 1/4 cup mixed berries
- Honey or maple syrup for sweetness (optional)

Instructions:

1. Cook oats with almond milk until creamy.
2. Top with nuts, berries, and sweetener if desired.

Veggie Omelette

Ingredients:

- 2 eggs
- 1/4 cup diced bell peppers and onions
- 1/4 cup sliced mushrooms
- Salt and pepper to taste

Instructions:

1. Whisk eggs in a bowl and season.
2. Cook the vegetables in a non-stick pan until tender.
3. Pour eggs over the veggies and cook until set. Fold in half and serve.

Whole Grain Pancakes

Ingredients:

- 1 cup whole grain pancake mix
- 1/2 cup water

- 1/4 cup fresh blueberries

Instructions:

1. Mix pancake batter with water.
2. Cook pancakes and add blueberries.
3. Serve with a drizzle of honey.

Chia Seed Pudding

Ingredients:

- 2 tablespoons chia seeds
- 1 cup unsweetened almond milk
- 1/2 teaspoon vanilla extract
- 1 tablespoon honey
- Fresh fruit for topping (e.g., berries, sliced banana)

Instructions:

1. In a jar, mix chia seeds, almond milk, vanilla, and honey.
2. Stir well, cover, and refrigerate overnight.
3. In the morning, top with your favorite fresh fruits.

Breakfast Burrito

Ingredients:

- 2 whole-grain tortillas
- 4 egg whites
- 1/4 cup black beans
- 1/4 cup diced bell peppers and onions
- Salsa (optional)

Instructions:

1. Scramble egg whites and cook with vegetables.
2. Warm tortillas in a dry pan.
3. Fill tortillas with eggs, black beans, and salsa.
4. Roll up and enjoy your burrito.

Almond Butter Toast

Ingredients:

- 2 slices of whole-grain bread
- 2 tablespoons almond butter
- Sliced banana or strawberries for topping

Instructions:

1. Toast the bread to your preference.

2. Spread almond butter and top with fruit slices.

3. A simple yet satisfying breakfast.

Smoothie Bowl

Ingredients:

- 1 cup unsweetened Greek yogurt

- 1/2 cup mixed berries

- 1 small banana

- 2 tablespoons honey

- Toppings: granola, nuts, or more fruit

Instructions:

1. Blend yogurt, berries, banana, and honey until smooth.

2. Pour into a bowl and add your choice of toppings.

Avocado Toast

Ingredients:

- 2 slices of whole-grain bread

- 1 ripe avocado

- Salt, pepper, and red pepper flakes to taste

Instructions:

1. Toast the bread.

2. Mash avocado and spread on the toast.

3. Season with salt, pepper, and a dash of red pepper flakes.

Cottage Cheese Pancakes

Ingredients:

- 1 cup low-fat cottage cheese

- 2 eggs

- 1/4 cup whole wheat flour

- 1/2 teaspoon vanilla extract

- Fresh berries for topping

Instructions:

1. In a blender, combine cottage cheese, eggs, whole wheat flour, and vanilla extract until smooth.

2. Heat a non-stick pan and cook small pancakes from the mixture.

3. Top with fresh berries.

Quinoa Porridge

Ingredients:

- 1/2 cup quinoa
- 1 cup almond milk
- 1/4 cup chopped nuts (e.g., almonds, walnuts)
- 1/4 cup dried fruits (e.g., raisins, apricots)
- A drizzle of honey or maple syrup

Instructions:

1. Rinse quinoa and cook it in almond milk until soft and creamy.
2. Top with chopped nuts, dried fruits, and a drizzle of sweetener.

Veggie Frittata

Ingredients:

- 4 eggs
- 1/2 cup chopped mixed vegetables (e.g., bell peppers, spinach, mushrooms)

- 1/4 cup grated low-fat cheese
- Salt and pepper to taste

Instructions:

1. Whisk eggs and season with salt and pepper.
2. Cook vegetables in an oven-safe skillet until tender.
3. Pour eggs over the veggies and sprinkle with cheese.
4. Bake in the oven until set and lightly golden.

Breakfast Quiche

Ingredients:

- 1 whole wheat pie crust
- 4 eggs
- 1/2 cup skim milk
- 1 cup diced vegetables (e.g., broccoli, tomatoes, onions)
- 1/2 cup low-fat cheese

Instructions:

1. Preheat the oven and bake the pie crust until lightly browned.

2. Whisk eggs and milk, then stir in vegetables and cheese.

3. Pour this mixture into the crust and bake until set.

Berry Smoothie

Ingredients:

- 1/2 cup mixed berries (e.g., strawberries, blueberries, raspberries)
- 1 cup unsweetened almond milk
- 1/2 banana
- 2 tablespoons Greek yogurt
- 1 tablespoon honey (optional)

Instructions:

1. Blend berries, almond milk, banana, Greek yogurt, and honey until smooth.

2. Enjoy this refreshing smoothie for a quick and healthy start to your day.

Chapter 3: Lunch Recipes

These recipes are not just for those with diabetes but for anyone looking to enjoy a wholesome and balanced midday meal. With a mix of protein-packed dishes and veggie-loaded options, you'll find something here to suit your taste and dietary needs.

Grilled Chicken Salad

Ingredients:

- Boneless, skinless chicken breasts
- Mixed salad greens
- Cherry tomatoes
- Cucumber
- Red onion
- Olive oil
- Balsamic vinegar
- Salt and pepper

Instructions:

1. Season chicken with salt and pepper.

2. Grill the chicken until cooked through.

3. Slice the chicken and serve it over mixed greens with cherry tomatoes, cucumber, and red onion.

4. Drizzle with a mix of olive oil and balsamic vinegar.

Lentil Soup

Ingredients:

- Green or brown lentils
- Onion
- Carrots
- Celery
- Garlic
- Vegetable broth
- Bay leaves
- Cumin
- Salt and pepper

Instructions:

1. Sauté chopped onions, carrots, and celery in a pot until softened.

2. Add garlic, lentils, vegetable broth, bay leaves, and cumin.

3. Simmer until lentils are tender, and season with salt
   and pepper.

Quinoa Salad

Ingredients:

- Quinoa
- Cucumber
- Red bell pepper
- Red onion
- Fresh parsley
- Olive oil
- Lemon juice
- Salt and pepper

Instructions:

1. Cook quinoa according to package instructions and
   let it cool.
2. Combine quinoa with chopped cucumber, red bell
   pepper, red onion, and fresh parsley.
3. Drizzle with olive oil and lemon juice, then season
   with salt and pepper.

Tuna Lettuce Wraps

Ingredients:

- Canned tuna
- Celery
- Red onion
- Mayonnaise
- Dill
- Lettuce leaves

Instructions:

1. Mix drained tuna with chopped celery, red onion, mayonnaise, and dill.
2. Spoon the tuna mixture into lettuce leaves and wrap them up.

Turkey and Avocado Wrap

Ingredients:

- Whole-grain tortilla
- Sliced turkey
- Avocado
- Spinach leaves

- Greek yogurt
- Mustard

Instructions:

1. Lay out a tortilla and layer with turkey, avocado, spinach, Greek yogurt, and a touch of mustard.
2. Roll it up and cut in half.

Spinach and Chickpea Salad

Ingredients:

- Fresh spinach
- Chickpeas
- Cherry tomatoes
- Red onion
- Feta cheese
- Balsamic vinaigrette

Instructions:

1. Toss together fresh spinach, chickpeas, halved cherry tomatoes, red onion, and crumbled feta cheese.
2. Drizzle with balsamic vinaigrette.

Cucumber and Hummus Sandwich

Ingredients:

- Whole-grain bread
- Hummus
- Cucumber
- Red bell pepper
- Sprouts

Instructions:

1. Spread hummus on whole-grain bread.
2. Add cucumber, red bell pepper, and sprouts for a refreshing sandwich.

Salmon and Asparagus

Ingredients:

- Salmon fillets
- Asparagus spears
- Lemon
- Olive oil
- Garlic
- Dill

Instructions:

1. Drizzle salmon and asparagus with olive oil, lemon juice, and minced garlic.

2. Season with dill and bake until the salmon flakes and asparagus is tender.

Spinach and Feta Stuffed Chicken Breast

Ingredients:

- Chicken breasts
- Spinach
- Feta cheese
- Garlic
- Olive oil
- Paprika
- Salt and pepper

Instructions:

1. Cut a pocket in each chicken breast.

2. Stuff with a mixture of spinach, feta, and garlic.

3. Rub with olive oil, paprika, salt, and pepper.

4. Bake until chicken is cooked through.

Black Bean and Quinoa Bowl

Ingredients:

- Cooked quinoa
- Black beans
- Corn
- Bell peppers
- Red onion
- Lime juice
- Cilantro
- Cumin
- Chili powder
- Salt and pepper

Instructions:

1. Mix cooked quinoa with black beans, corn, diced bell peppers, and red onion.
2. Toss with a dressing of lime juice, cilantro, cumin, chili powder, salt, and pepper.

Shrimp and Vegetable Stir-Fry

Ingredients:

- Shrimp
- Broccoli florets
- Bell peppers
- Snap peas
- Ginger
- Garlic
- Soy sauce
- Sesame oil
- Rice vinegar

Instructions:

1. Sauté shrimp in sesame oil with ginger and garlic.
2. Add broccoli, bell peppers, and snap peas, stir-fry until tender.
3. Finish with a sauce made from soy sauce and rice vinegar.

Egg Salad Lettuce Wraps

Ingredients:

- Hard-boiled eggs
- Greek yogurt
- Dijon mustard
- Celery
- Chives
- Lettuce leaves

Instructions:

1. Chop hard-boiled eggs and mix with Greek yogurt, Dijon mustard, celery, and chives.
2. Spoon the egg salad into lettuce leaves and serve.

Cauliflower Rice Bowl

Ingredients:

- Cauliflower rice
- Ground turkey
- Bell peppers
- Zucchini
- Olive oil

- Paprika

- Cumin

- Salt and pepper

Instructions:

1. Sauté ground turkey with diced bell peppers and zucchini.

2. Add cauliflower rice and season with olive oil, paprika, cumin, salt, and pepper.

Caprese Salad

Ingredients:

- Tomato slices

- Fresh mozzarella slices

- Fresh basil leaves

- Balsamic glaze

- Olive oil

- Salt and pepper

Instructions:

1. Arrange tomato and mozzarella slices with fresh basil.

2. Drizzle with olive oil and balsamic glaze, then season with salt and pepper.

Sweet Potato and Black Bean Quesadilla

Ingredients:

- Whole-grain tortilla
- Sweet potato
- Black beans
- Red onion
- Cumin
- Paprika
- Olive oil
- Greek yogurt

Instructions:

1. Roast sweet potato with olive oil, cumin, and paprika.
2. Mash the black beans and spread them on a tortilla.
3. Add roasted sweet potato, diced red onion, and a dollop of Greek yogurt.

4.   Fold the tortilla in half and cook until crispy.

Chapter 4: Dinner Recipes

In this chapter, we're delighted to present a collection of delicious dinner recipes designed to keep your blood sugar stable while tantalizing your taste buds. These low glycemic index options offer a variety of flavors and ingredients, making it easier to stick to your dietary goals.

Baked Salmon with Dill

Ingredients:

- 4 salmon fillets
- 2 tablespoons fresh dill
- 1 lemon, sliced
- Salt and pepper to taste

Instructions:

1. Preheat your oven to 375°F (190°C).
2. Place salmon fillets on a baking sheet.
3. Sprinkle fresh dill over the salmon.
4. Lay lemon slices on top.
5. Season with salt and pepper.

6. Bake for 15-20 minutes or until the salmon flakes easily with a fork.

Chicken and Broccoli Stir-Fry

Ingredients:

- 2 boneless, skinless chicken breasts, cubed
- 2 cups broccoli florets
- 1/4 cup low-sodium soy sauce
- 2 cloves garlic, minced
- 1 tablespoon ginger, minced

Instructions:

1. Heat a non-stick pan over medium heat.
2. Add chicken and cook until no longer pink.
3. Add broccoli, soy sauce, garlic, and ginger.
4. Stir-fry until the broccoli is tender and the chicken is cooked through.

Spinach and Mushroom Stuffed Pork Tenderloin

Ingredients:

- 1 pork tenderloin
- 2 cups fresh spinach
- 1 cup mushrooms, sliced
- 2 cloves garlic, minced
- Salt and pepper to taste

Instructions:

1. Preheat your oven to 375°F (190°C).
2. Butterfly the pork tenderloin and season with salt and pepper.
3. Sauté mushrooms and garlic in a pan until soft.
4. Lay spinach over the pork, followed by the mushroom mixture.
5. Roll up the tenderloin and secure with toothpicks.
6. Bake for 25-30 minutes or until the pork is cooked through.

Grilled Vegetable Plate

Ingredients:

- An assortment of your favorite low GI vegetables (e.g., zucchini, bell peppers, eggplant)
- Olive oil
- Herbs and spices of your choice

Instructions:

1. Slice vegetables into even pieces.
2. Brush with olive oil and season with herbs and spices.
3. Grill until tender and slightly charred.

Beef and Snow Pea Stir-Fry

Ingredients:

- 1 pound lean beef, thinly sliced
- 2 cups snow peas
- 2 tablespoons low-sodium soy sauce
- 1 tablespoon oyster sauce
- 2 cloves garlic, minced

Instructions:

1. Heat a wok or large pan over high heat.

2. Stir-fry beef until browned. Set aside.

3. In the same pan, stir-fry snow peas and garlic for a few minutes.

4. Return the beef and add soy sauce and oyster sauce.

5. Cook until everything is heated through.

Lemon Herb Baked Tilapia

Ingredients:

- 4 tilapia fillets
- Zest and juice of 1 lemon
- 2 tablespoons fresh herbs (e.g., thyme, rosemary)
- Salt and pepper to taste

Instructions:

1. Preheat your oven to 375°F (190°C).

2. Place tilapia fillets on a baking sheet.

3. Sprinkle with lemon zest, lemon juice, and herbs.

4. Season with salt and pepper.

5. Bake for about 15-20 minutes until the fish flakes easily.

Turkey and Quinoa Stuffed Bell Peppers

Ingredients:

- 4 bell peppers
- 1 cup cooked quinoa
- 1 pound ground turkey
- 1 cup tomato sauce
- 1/2 cup shredded low-fat cheese

Instructions:

1. Preheat your oven to 375°F (190°C).
2. Cut the tops off the bell peppers and remove seeds.
3. In a pan, brown the ground turkey.
4. Combine cooked quinoa and half of the tomato sauce with the turkey.
5. Stuff the bell peppers with the mixture.
6. Place the stuffed peppers in a baking dish, pour the remaining tomato sauce over them, and sprinkle with cheese.
7. Bake for 20-25 minutes.

Spaghetti Squash with Pesto

Ingredients:

- 1 spaghetti squash
- 1/2 cup basil pesto
- Cherry tomatoes for garnish
- Grated Parmesan cheese (optional)

Instructions:

1. Preheat your oven to 375°F (190°C).
2. Cut the spaghetti squash in half lengthwise and remove seeds.
3. Roast the squash halves in the oven for 30-40 minutes.
4. Use a fork to scrape out the "spaghetti" strands.
5. Toss with pesto, garnish with cherry tomatoes, and add Parmesan cheese if desired.

Cabbage and Turkey Sauté

Ingredients:

- 1 pound ground turkey
- 1 small cabbage, thinly sliced

- 1 onion, chopped
- 2 cloves garlic, minced
- 1 tablespoon olive oil
- Salt and pepper to taste

Instructions:

1. In a large skillet, heat olive oil over medium heat.
2. Add chopped onion and garlic, sauté until fragrant.
3. Add ground turkey and cook until browned.
4. Stir in sliced cabbage and cook until it wilts and becomes tender.
5. Season with salt and pepper.

Baked Cod with Asparagus

Ingredients:

- 4 cod fillets
- 1 bunch of asparagus
- 2 tablespoons lemon juice
- 2 cloves garlic, minced
- Fresh dill for garnish
- Salt and pepper to taste

Instructions:

1. Preheat your oven to 375°F (190°C).

2. Place cod fillets and asparagus on a baking sheet.

3. Drizzle with lemon juice and sprinkle with garlic, dill, salt, and pepper.

4. Bake for about 15-20 minutes until the cod flakes easily.

Chicken and Zucchini Skewers

Ingredients:

- 2 boneless, skinless chicken breasts, cubed
- 2 zucchinis, sliced into rounds
- 1 red onion, cut into chunks
- Olive oil
- Lemon zest
- Your choice of herbs and spices

Instructions:

1. Preheat your grill.

2. Thread chicken, zucchini, and onion onto skewers.

3. Brush with olive oil and season with lemon zest, herbs, and spices.

4. Grill until the chicken is cooked through and the vegetables are tender.

Quinoa and Black Bean Stuffed Peppers

Ingredients:

- 4 bell peppers
- 1 cup cooked quinoa
- 1 cup black beans
- 1 cup diced tomatoes
- 1 teaspoon cumin
- 1/2 cup low-fat cheese for topping

Instructions:

1. Preheat your oven to 375°F (190°C).
2. Cut the tops off the bell peppers and remove seeds.
3. In a bowl, mix quinoa, black beans, diced tomatoes, and cumin.
4. Stuff the bell peppers with the mixture.
5. Sprinkle with cheese.
6. Bake for 20-25 minutes.

Seared Tofu with Vegetables

Ingredients:

- 1 block of firm tofu, cubed
- An assortment of your favorite low GI vegetables
- Low-sodium soy sauce
- Sesame oil
- Minced garlic and ginger

Instructions:

1. Heat a skillet over medium-high heat.
2. Sear tofu until golden brown on all sides.
3. Add your choice of vegetables and stir-fry.
4. Season with soy sauce, sesame oil, garlic, and ginger.

Shrimp Scampi

Ingredients:

- 1 pound shrimp, peeled and deveined
- 2 tablespoons olive oil
- 3 cloves garlic, minced
- Juice of 1 lemon
- Chopped fresh parsley

- Salt and pepper to taste

Instructions:

1. In a skillet, heat olive oil over medium-high heat.
2. Add garlic and shrimp, sauté until shrimp turn pink.
3. Stir in lemon juice, parsley, salt, and pepper.

Vegetable Curry

Ingredients:

- Assorted vegetables (e.g., broccoli, cauliflower, carrots)
- 1 can of low-sodium chickpeas
- 1 can of coconut milk
- 2 tablespoons curry paste
- Fresh cilantro for garnish

Instructions:

1. In a large pot, combine vegetables, chickpeas, coconut milk, and curry paste.
2. Simmer until vegetables are tender and the sauce thickens.
3. Garnish with fresh cilantro.

Chapter 5: Snacks and Appetizers

In this chapter, we've curated a collection of snacks and appetizers that not only cater to your taste buds but also keep your blood sugar in check. These snacks are perfect for a midday pick-me-up or for entertaining guests. Let's dive into these delectable and diabetes-friendly snack recipes.

Guacamole with Veggie Sticks

Ingredients:

- 2 ripe avocados
- 1 small red onion, finely diced
- 1-2 tomatoes, diced
- 1 lime, juiced
- Salt and pepper to taste
- Assorted vegetable sticks (carrots, celery, bell peppers) for dipping

Instructions:

1. Cut the avocados in half, remove the pits, and scoop the flesh into a bowl.

2. Mash the avocados with a fork until you reach your desired consistency.

3. Add the diced onion, tomatoes, lime juice, salt, and pepper. Mix well.

4. Serve with a colorful array of vegetable sticks for dipping.

Roasted Chickpeas

Ingredients:

- 2 cans of chickpeas, drained and rinsed
- 2 tablespoons olive oil
- 1 teaspoon paprika
- 1/2 teaspoon cayenne pepper (adjust to taste)
- Salt to taste

Instructions:

1. Preheat your oven to 400°F (200°C).

2. Rinse and drain the chickpeas, then pat them dry with a paper towel.

3. In a bowl, toss the chickpeas with olive oil, paprika, cayenne pepper, and salt.

4. Spread them on a baking sheet and roast for about 30-40 minutes or until crispy.

Cottage Cheese and Pineapple

Ingredients:

- Low-fat cottage cheese
- Fresh pineapple chunks

Instructions:

1. Simply serve a portion of low-fat cottage cheese with fresh pineapple chunks for a refreshing and satisfying snack.

Edamame

Ingredients:

- Edamame pods
- Salt

Instructions:

1. Boil the edamame pods in salted water for 3-5 minutes.

2. Drain and let them cool slightly before enjoying.

Hummus and Whole Grain Crackers

Ingredients:

- Store-bought or homemade hummus
- Whole grain crackers

Instructions:

1. Serve hummus with whole grain crackers for a delightful combination of flavors and textures.

Greek Salad Skewers

Ingredients:

- Cherry tomatoes
- Cucumber slices
- Kalamata olives
- Feta cheese cubes
- Fresh basil leaves
- Balsamic vinaigrette for drizzling

Instructions:

1. Assemble the ingredients on skewers, creating a mini Greek salad on a stick.

2. Drizzle with balsamic vinaigrette before serving.

Avocado Slices with Salsa

Ingredients:

- Ripe avocados
- Salsa (store-bought or homemade)

Instructions:

1. Slice ripe avocados and serve with a side of salsa for dipping.

Deviled Eggs

Ingredients:

- Hard-boiled eggs
- Greek yogurt or mayonnaise
- Dijon mustard
- Paprika
- Chopped chives (optional)

Instructions:

1. Halve the hard-boiled eggs and remove the yolks.
2. Mix the yolks with Greek yogurt or mayonnaise, Dijon mustard, and a pinch of paprika.
3. Spoon the mixture back into the egg whites.
4. Garnish with chopped chives if desired.

Zucchini Chips

Ingredients:

- Zucchini, thinly sliced
- Olive oil
- Seasoning of your choice (try paprika or garlic powder)

Instructions:

1. Preheat your oven to 225°F (110°C).
2. Toss the zucchini slices in olive oil and your chosen seasoning.
3. Arrange them on a baking sheet and bake for 2-3 hours until crispy.

Cucumber Rolls with Cream Cheese

Ingredients:

- Cucumber, thinly sliced lengthwise
- Light cream cheese
- Fresh dill or chives for garnish

Instructions:

1. Lay out cucumber slices and spread a thin layer of light cream cheese on each slice.
2. Roll the cucumber slices and secure with a toothpick.
3. Garnish with fresh dill or chives.

Caprese Skewers

Ingredients:

- Cherry tomatoes
- Fresh mozzarella balls
- Fresh basil leaves
- Balsamic glaze for drizzling

Instructions:

1. Assemble cherry tomatoes, fresh mozzarella balls, and fresh basil leaves on skewers.
2. Drizzle with balsamic glaze for a burst of flavor.

Mixed Nuts

Ingredients:

- Assorted unsalted nuts (almonds, walnuts, cashews, etc.)

Instructions:

1. Create your own mix of unsalted nuts for a quick and satisfying snack.

Seaweed Snacks

Ingredients:

- Seaweed sheets

Instructions:

1. Enjoy store-bought seaweed snacks or make your own by toasting seaweed sheets with a dash of salt.

Baked Sweet Potato Fries

Ingredients:

- Sweet potatoes, cut into fries
- Olive oil
- Seasoning of your choice (try rosemary or garlic powder)

Instructions:

1. Preheat your oven to 425°F (220°C).
2. Toss sweet potato fries in olive oil and your preferred seasoning.
3. Bake for 20-30 minutes, flipping them halfway through, until they're crispy and golden.

Mini Meatballs with Dipping Sauce

Ingredients:

- Lean ground turkey or beef
- Bread crumbs (or almond meal for a low-carb option)
- Egg
- Minced garlic
- Salt and pepper

- Dipping sauce of your choice (try a sugar-free BBQ or tomato sauce)

Instructions:

1. In a bowl, mix the ground meat, bread crumbs, egg, minced garlic, salt, and pepper.
2. Roll the mixture into mini meatballs.
3. Bake or cook the meatballs as desired.
4. Serve with your favorite dipping sauce.

Chapter 6: Desserts

Here, we've crafted delectable, low glycemic index desserts to satisfy your sweet cravings without causing blood sugar spikes. Each recipe is thoughtfully designed, and we've provided the ingredients and step-by-step instructions to make it easy for you to enjoy guilt-free sweet treats.

Berry and Yogurt Parfait

Ingredients:

- 1 cup Greek yogurt
- 1/2 cup mixed berries (strawberries, blueberries, raspberries)
- 1 tablespoon honey
- 1/4 cup granola (optional)

Instructions:

1. In a glass, layer Greek yogurt, mixed berries, and honey.
2. Repeat the layers.
3. Top with granola for some added crunch if desired.

Dark Chocolate-Covered Strawberries

Ingredients:

- 8-10 fresh strawberries
- 2 oz dark chocolate (70% cocoa or higher)

Instructions:

1. Melt dark chocolate in a microwave-safe bowl.
2. Dip each strawberry into the melted chocolate.
3. Place on parchment paper and let it cool until the chocolate hardens.

Greek Yogurt with Honey and Walnuts

Ingredients:

- 1 cup Greek yogurt
- 1 tablespoon honey
- 2 tablespoons chopped walnuts

Instructions:

1. In a bowl, mix Greek yogurt and honey.

2. Sprinkle chopped walnuts on top before serving.

Sugar-Free Apple Crisp

Ingredients:

- 4 apples, peeled and sliced
- 1 cup almond flour
- 1/2 cup rolled oats
- 1/4 cup melted coconut oil
- 1 teaspoon cinnamon
- 1/4 teaspoon nutmeg
- 2 tablespoons sweetener (stevia or erythritol)

Instructions:

1. Preheat your oven to 350°F (175°C).
2. In a bowl, mix almond flour, rolled oats, melted coconut oil, cinnamon, nutmeg, and sweetener.
3. Place sliced apples in a baking dish and cover with the oat mixture.
4. Bake for 30-35 minutes until the topping is golden and the apples are tender.

Baked Pears with Cinnamon

Ingredients:

- 2 ripe pears, halved and cored
- 1 teaspoon cinnamon
- 2 teaspoons honey

Instructions:

1. Preheat your oven to 350°F (175°C).
2. Place pear halves in a baking dish.
3. Sprinkle cinnamon and drizzle honey over the pears.
4. Bake for about 25-30 minutes until pears are tender and caramelized.

Avocado Chocolate Mousse

Ingredients:

- 2 ripe avocados
- 1/4 cup unsweetened cocoa powder
- 1/4 cup almond milk
- 3 tablespoons honey
- 1 teaspoon vanilla extract

Instructions:

1. In a food processor, blend avocados, cocoa powder, almond milk, honey, and vanilla extract until smooth.
2. Chill in the refrigerator for at least 30 minutes before serving.

Chia Seed Chocolate Pudding

Ingredients:

- 3 tablespoons chia seeds
- 1 cup unsweetened almond milk
- 2 tablespoons unsweetened cocoa powder
- 1 tablespoon honey
- 1/2 teaspoon vanilla extract

Instructions:

1. In a bowl, whisk chia seeds, almond milk, cocoa powder, honey, and vanilla extract.
2. Refrigerate for at least 2 hours, stirring occasionally, until it thickens.

Coconut Macaroons

Ingredients:

- 2 cups unsweetened shredded coconut
- 1/2 cup egg whites
- 1/4 cup honey
- 1/2 teaspoon vanilla extract

Instructions:

1. Preheat your oven to 350°F (175°C).
2. In a bowl, mix shredded coconut, egg whites, honey, and vanilla extract.
3. Drop spoonfuls of the mixture onto a baking sheet.
4. Bake for 15-20 minutes until golden brown.

Raspberry Sorbet

Ingredients:

- 2 cups frozen raspberries
- 1/4 cup unsweetened almond milk
- 2 tablespoons honey
- 1 teaspoon lemon juice

Instructions:

1. In a blender, combine frozen raspberries, almond milk, honey, and lemon juice.
2. Blend until smooth and serve immediately.

Almond and Blueberry Bites

Ingredients:

- 1/2 cup almond butter
- 1/4 cup almond meal
- 1/4 cup dried blueberries
- 1 tablespoon honey

Instructions:

1. In a bowl, mix almond butter, almond meal, dried blueberries, and honey.
2. Roll the mixture into small bites and refrigerate.

Lemon Poppy Seed Cake

Ingredients:

- 1 cup almond flour
- 1/4 cup coconut flour

- 2 tablespoons poppy seeds

- 1/4 cup lemon juice

- 1/4 cup honey

- 1/4 cup unsweetened almond milk

- 1/2 teaspoon baking powder

- Zest from 1 lemon

Instructions:

1. Preheat your oven to 350°F (175°C).

2. In a bowl, combine almond flour, coconut flour, poppy seeds, baking powder, and lemon zest.

3. In another bowl, whisk together lemon juice, honey, and almond milk.

4. Mix the wet ingredients into the dry ingredients.

5. Pour the batter into a greased cake pan and bake for 25-30 minutes, or until a toothpick comes out clean.

Peanut Butter Protein Balls

Ingredients:

- 1 cup natural peanut butter

- 1/2 cup whey protein powder

- 1/4 cup ground flaxseed

- 2 tablespoons honey
- 1/2 teaspoon vanilla extract

Instructions:

1. In a bowl, combine peanut butter, whey protein powder, ground flaxseed, honey, and vanilla extract.
2. Roll the mixture into small balls and refrigerate.

Vanilla and Almond Milkshake

Ingredients:

- 1 cup unsweetened almond milk
- 1/2 teaspoon vanilla extract
- 2 tablespoons unsweetened almond butter
- 1/2 teaspoon honey (or a sugar substitute)

Instructions:

1. In a blender, combine almond milk, vanilla extract, almond butter, and honey.
2. Blend until smooth and creamy.

Pumpkin Pie Smoothie

Ingredients:

- 1/2 cup pumpkin puree
- 1 cup unsweetened almond milk
- 1/2 teaspoon pumpkin pie spice
- 1/2 teaspoon cinnamon
- 1/2 teaspoon honey (optional)

Instructions:

1. In a blender, combine pumpkin puree, almond milk, pumpkin pie spice, cinnamon, and honey (if desired).
2. Blend until smooth.

Banana Walnut Ice Cream

Ingredients:

- 2 ripe bananas, sliced and frozen
- 1/4 cup chopped walnuts
- 1/2 teaspoon vanilla extract

Instructions:

1. Place frozen banana slices in a food processor.

2. Add chopped walnuts and vanilla extract.

3. Process until it reaches a creamy ice cream consistency.

Chapter 7: Smoothies

These smoothie recipes have been thoughtfully crafted to be both low in glycemic index and bursting with flavor. Enjoy a variety of ingredients that not only taste great but also help keep your blood sugar levels in check.

Green Spinach Smoothie

Ingredients:

- 1 cup fresh spinach leaves
- 1/2 cucumber, peeled and sliced
- 1 green apple, cored and chopped
- 1/2 lemon, juiced
- 1/2 cup water
- Ice cubes (optional)

Instructions:

1. Place all the ingredients in a blender.
2. Blend until smooth.
3. Add ice cubes if desired.
4. Pour into a glass and enjoy!

Berry Blast Smoothie

Ingredients:

- 1/2 cup mixed berries (strawberries, blueberries, raspberries)
- 1/2 cup plain Greek yogurt
- 1/2 banana
- 1 tablespoon honey (optional)
- 1/2 cup water or unsweetened almond milk

Instructions:

1. Combine all the ingredients in a blender.
2. Blend until you achieve a smooth, creamy texture.
3. Sweeten with honey if needed.
4. Serve and savor the berry goodness!

Mango Tango Smoothie

Ingredients:

- 1 ripe mango, peeled and diced
- 1/2 cup plain yogurt
- 1/2 cup unsweetened almond milk
- 1/2 teaspoon vanilla extract

- 1/2 teaspoon ground cinnamon
- Ice cubes (optional)

Instructions:

1. Put all the ingredients in a blender.
2. Blend until the mixture is velvety smooth.
3. Add ice if you prefer it chilled.
4. Pour into a glass and indulge in the tropical vibes.

Peanut Butter Banana Smoothie

Ingredients:

- 1 ripe banana
- 2 tablespoons natural peanut butter
- 1/2 cup plain Greek yogurt
- 1/2 cup unsweetened almond milk
- 1 tablespoon flaxseeds (optional)

Instructions:

1. Place all ingredients in a blender.
2. Blend until creamy and smooth.
3. Add flaxseeds for an extra boost.
4. Pour into a glass and enjoy the nutty sweetness.

Almond Joy Smoothie

Ingredients:

- 1/2 cup unsweetened almond milk
- 1/4 cup shredded unsweetened coconut
- 1 tablespoon unsweetened cocoa powder
- 1/4 teaspoon almond extract
- 1/2 ripe banana
- Ice cubes (optional)

Instructions:

1. Blend all the ingredients until well combined.
2. Add ice for a chilled, refreshing twist.
3. Pour into a glass and savor the taste of an almond joy.

Spinach and Pineapple Smoothie

Ingredients:

- 1 cup fresh spinach leaves
- 1/2 cup pineapple chunks
- 1/2 banana
- 1/2 cup coconut water
- 1 tablespoon chia seeds (optional)

Instructions:

1. Place the ingredients in a blender.

2. Blend until you have a smooth consistency.

3. Add chia seeds for extra nutrition.

4. Serve up this tropical green delight.

Chocolate Protein Shake

Ingredients:

- 1 cup unsweetened almond milk
- 1 scoop chocolate protein powder
- 1 tablespoon unsweetened cocoa powder
- 1/2 banana
- Ice cubes (optional)

Instructions:

1. Blend all the ingredients until creamy and well-mixed.

2. Add ice for a frosty finish.

3. Enjoy this protein-packed chocolate treat.

Kiwi and Kale Smoothie

Ingredients:

- 1 ripe kiwi, peeled and sliced
- 1 cup fresh kale leaves
- 1/2 banana
- 1/2 cup plain Greek yogurt
- 1/2 cup water

Instructions:

1. Combine the ingredients in a blender.
2. Blend until you achieve a smooth texture.
3. Pour into a glass and relish the green goodness.

Blueberry and Avocado Smoothie

Ingredients:

- 1/2 cup blueberries
- 1/4 ripe avocado
- 1/2 cup plain yogurt
- 1/2 cup unsweetened almond milk
- 1 tablespoon honey (optional)

Instructions:

1. Place all the ingredients in a blender.
2. Blend until creamy and luscious.
3. Sweeten with honey if desired.
4. Enjoy the unique blend of blueberries and avocado.

Strawberry and Oatmeal Smoothie

Ingredients:

- 1/2 cup fresh strawberries
- 1/4 cup rolled oats
- 1/2 cup plain Greek yogurt
- 1/2 cup unsweetened almond milk
- 1 teaspoon honey (optional)

Instructions:

1. Blend all ingredients until smooth.
2. Sweeten with honey if desired.
3. Pour into a glass and enjoy a wholesome breakfast in a glass.

Coconut Chia Smoothie

Ingredients:

- 1/2 cup coconut milk
- 2 tablespoons chia seeds
- 1/2 banana
- 1/2 cup fresh pineapple chunks
- Ice cubes (optional)

Instructions:

1. Combine the ingredients in a blender.
2. Blend until you have a rich, creamy mixture.
3. Add ice cubes for a refreshing twist.
4. Sip on this tropical delight.

Spinach and Apple Smoothie

Ingredients:

- 1 cup fresh spinach leaves
- 1 apple, cored and sliced
- 1/2 cup plain Greek yogurt
- 1/2 cup unsweetened almond milk
- 1/2 teaspoon ground cinnamon

Instructions:

1. Place all ingredients in a blender.
2. Blend until you have a green, smooth consistency.
3. Savor the delightful blend of spinach and apple.

Peach and Almond Smoothie

Ingredients:

- 1 ripe peach, pitted and sliced
- 1/4 cup almonds
- 1/2 cup plain Greek yogurt
- 1/2 cup unsweetened almond milk
- 1 tablespoon honey (optional)

Instructions:

1. Combine all the ingredients in a blender.
2. Blend until creamy and nutty.
3. Sweeten with honey if desired.
4. Enjoy the taste of fresh peaches and almonds.

Tropical Paradise Smoothie

Ingredients:

- 1/2 cup fresh pineapple chunks
- 1/2 banana
- 1/2 cup coconut water
- 1/2 cup Greek yogurt
- Ice cubes (optional)

Instructions:

1. Place all ingredients in a blender.
2. Blend until you have a tropical paradise in a glass.
3. Add ice cubes for an extra refreshing kick.

Carrot and Ginger Smoothie

Ingredients:

- 1 carrot, peeled and sliced
- 1/2-inch piece of fresh ginger
- 1/2 cup plain Greek yogurt
- 1/2 cup water
- 1 tablespoon honey (optional)

Instructions:

1. Blend all the ingredients until smooth.

2. Sweeten with honey if desired.

3. Sip on this zesty and nutritious carrot and ginger blend.

CONCLUSION

In the final chapter of our journey towards healthier living with low glycemic index diabetic recipes, we wrap up with a sense of accomplishment and a wealth of knowledge at our fingertips. This chapter serves as a guide to take all the valuable insights from the preceding chapters and apply them in practical ways to lead a fulfilling life while managing diabetes.

1. **Reflecting on Your Progress:** We encourage you to pause and reflect on the path you've traveled so far. Celebrate your achievements, no matter how small they may seem. Remember, every step counts on this journey to better health.

2. **Sustaining Positive Habits:** Discover strategies to maintain the positive dietary and lifestyle changes you've adopted. Learn how to make these changes a permanent part of your life, ensuring long-term success in managing your diabetes.

3. **Community and Support:** Connecting with others who face similar challenges can be a tremendous

source of inspiration and encouragement. We explore ways to engage with support groups, both in person and online, to share experiences and gain insights.

4. **Self-Care and Mindfulness:** Caring for your mental and emotional well-being is equally important. We delve into the importance of self-care, stress management, and mindfulness, offering techniques to reduce the psychological burden of diabetes.

5. **Setting New Goals**: As one chapter closes, another begins. Set new health and wellness goals, adjusting them to your evolving needs and aspirations. We provide a framework for creating achievable goals and tracking your progress.

6. **The Bigger Picture:** Understanding how your journey contributes to a broader picture is crucial. We explore the impact of managing diabetes on your overall health and the potential for preventing complications in the long run.

In this concluding chapter, we emphasize that managing diabetes is not a one-time event but a lifelong journey. By taking the knowledge and tools gained from this book and continuing to apply them in your daily life, you can lead a fulfilling and healthy life while effectively managing your diabetes. Your story is unique, and with the right information and support, it's a story of triumph and vitality.